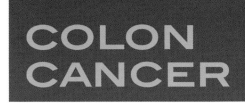

COLON CANCER

Current and Emerging Trends in Detection and Treatment

MARK STOKES, MD, FACP

The Rosen Publishing Group, Inc., New York

For Fiona

Published in 2006 by The Rosen Publishing Group, Inc.
29 East 21st Street, New York, NY 10010

Library of Congress Cataloging-in-Publication Data

Stokes, Mark.
Colon cancer: current and emerging trends in detection and treatment/
by Mark Stokes.—1st ed.
   p. cm.—(Cancer and modern science)
ISBN 1-4042-0387-7 (lib. bdg.)
1. Colon (Anatomy)—Cancer.
I. Title. II. Series.
RC280.C6S755 2006
616.99'4347—dc22

                                                    2005003626

Manufactured in Malaysia

On the cover: Scanning electron micrograph of human colon cancer cells, magnified
15,000 times the actual size.

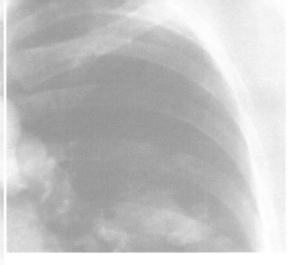

CONTENTS

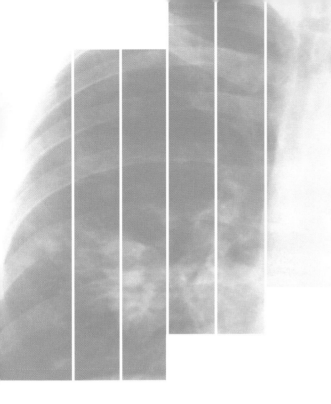

INTRODUCTION

What do baseball stars Darryl Strawberry and Eric Davis, Supreme Court Justice Ruth Bader Ginsberg, and music promoter and TV personality Sharon Osbourne have in common? They all have the diagnosis of colorectal cancer, which includes cancer of the colon and rectum. Each year, approximately 135,000 Americans are diagnosed with colorectal cancer. It is the third most common cancer in the United States, and it is the third leading cause of cancer death, at a rate of 60,000 per year. *Peanuts* creator Charles Schulz, comedian Milton Berle, and movie actresses Audrey Hepburn and Elizabeth Montgomery all died of colorectal cancer.

Unlike other cancers, such as those of the lung, prostate, and breast, colorectal cancer is preventable provided that the biology of the disease is understood and the appropriate screening tests are used. This is because colorectal cancer has a clearly recognized premalignant stage—a period during which damaged cells that could lead to cancer are not yet cancerous—whereas other cancers do not. By targeting treatment

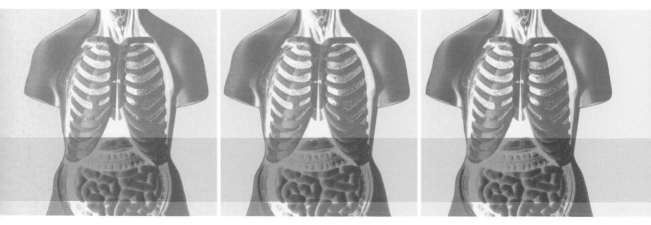

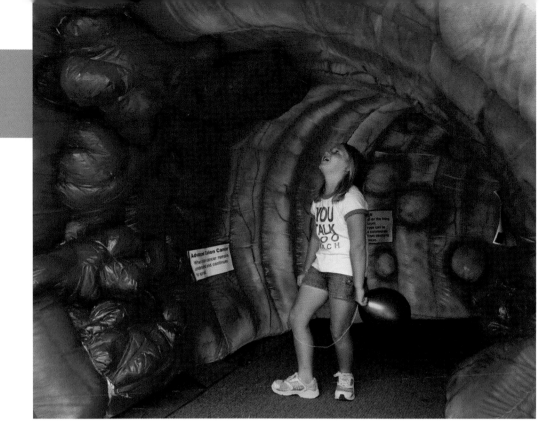

A young girl looks at a section of a twenty-foot-long (six-meter-long) model of a colon that portrays cancerous colon tissues. The model was the main feature of the Cancer Research and Prevention Foundation's "Check Your Insides Out from Top to Bottom" booth at the Oklahoma State Fair on September 21, 2004. Colon cancer awareness programs like these have multiplied across the United States in recent years.

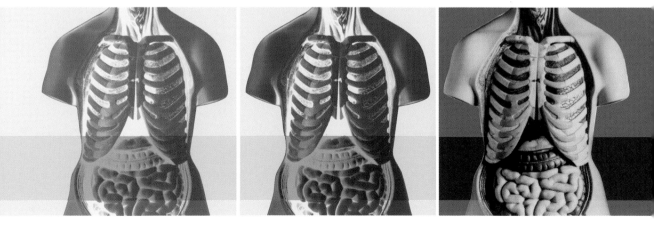

during this stage, colorectal cancer itself can be prevented. Moreover, because it is possible to identify who might have these premalignant lesions, the number of patients with colorectal cancer should be declining. Unfortunately it is not.

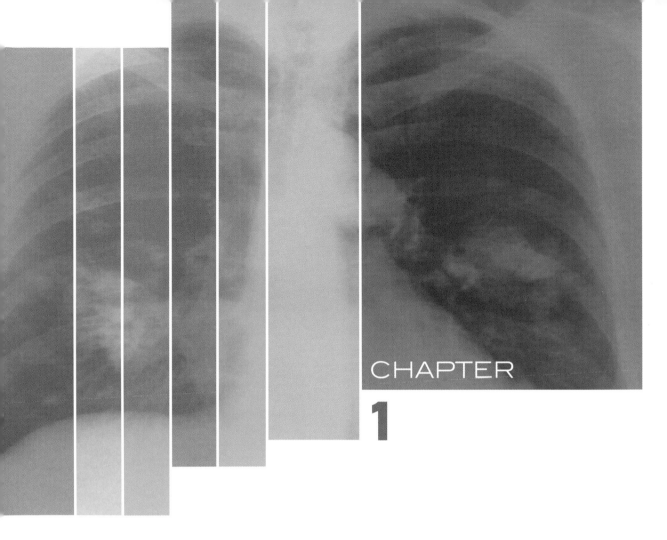

WHAT IS CANCER?

To understand the diagnosis and treatment of cancer, it is important to understand cancer itself. Cancer begins in cells, the smallest self-functioning units in all living things. Cells make up tissues, which make up the organs of the body. All cells contain specific genes that govern the number of times the cells reproduce. Cells reproduce by dividing themselves. When a cell has divided a determined number of times, it then ceases to divide further. Some genes also program cells to die when that number is reached.

A number of checks and balances take place within each cell to regulate this process of division. The development of cancer occurs when this system breaks down. When this happens, the genes that are involved in the growth-limiting attributes of the cell are damaged, allowing the cell to take on an immortal nature. In other words, the cancerous cell will divide indefinitely. Genes that render cells immortal are known as oncogenes (from the Greek words *onkos* for "mass" and *genea* for "generation"). They may once have been normal growth-regulating genes that became mutated. Some oncogenes may have existed all along but were kept inactive in the normal noncancerous state of the cell. They may have been turned on either by a mutation during the normal course of cell division or damaged by a carcinogen and were repaired improperly.

Once immortal, the cells grow unchecked, forming visible masses called tumors. Tumors can be benign or malignant. Benign tumors are noncancerous and are rarely life-threatening. Malignant tumors are cancerous, and they are often life-threatening because they can destroy the normal tissues of the body. Unlike the cells of benign tumors, malignant tumor cells can invade and damage nearby tissues and organs, as well as spread to other parts of the body. Cancer cells spread by breaking away from the primary tumor, or original cancer, and entering the bloodstream or the lymphatic system, which consists of the tissues and organs that produce and store cells that fight disease and infection. They then enter other organs, where they form new tumors, thus damaging the organs. The spread of cancer is called metastasis.

UNDERSTANDING COLON CANCER

Colon cancer is cancer that develops in the tissues of the colon. The colon is a part of the digestive system. Together with the rectum, it forms the large intestine, which is a long, muscular tube that measures 4 to 5 feet

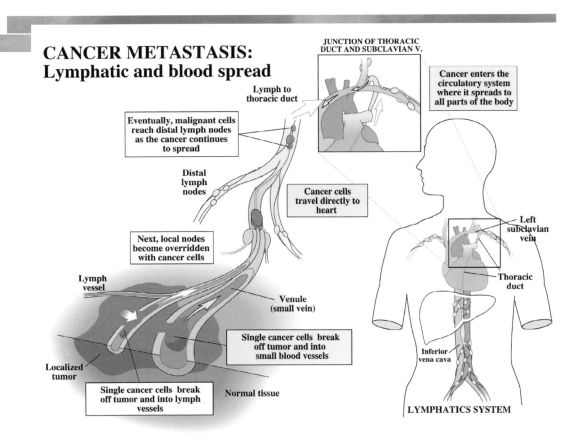

CANCER METASTASIS:
Lymphatic and blood spread

JUNCTION OF THORACIC DUCT AND SUBCLAVIAN V.

Cancer enters the circulatory system where it spreads to all parts of the body

Lymph to thoracic duct

Eventually, malignant cells reach distal lymph nodes as the cancer continues to spread

Distal lymph nodes

Cancer cells travel directly to heart

Next, local nodes become overridden with cancer cells

Left subclavian vein

Lymph vessel

Venule (small vein)

Thoracic duct

Single cancer cells break off tumor and into small blood vessels

Inferior vena cava

Localized tumor

Single cancer cells break off tumor and into lymph vessels

Normal tissue

LYMPHATICS SYSTEM

Metastasis occurs when cancerous cells break away from the original tumor, enter the bloodstream or the lymphatic system, and travel to other parts of the body.

(1.2 to 1.5 m). The part of the colon that connects it to the rectum is called the sigmoid colon. At its other end, the colon is connected to the small intestine at the cecum.

The colon performs an important bodily function. It removes water and nutrients from partially digested food that comes from the small

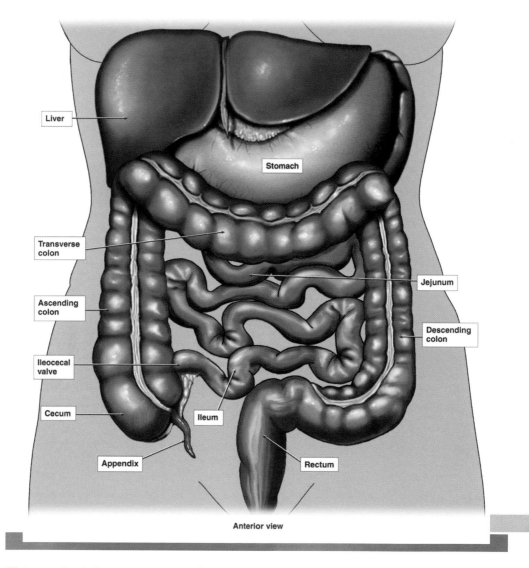

Liver

Stomach

Transverse colon

Jejunum

Ascending colon

Descending colon

Ileocecal valve

Cecum

Ileum

Appendix

Rectum

Anterior view

This medical illustration provides an anterior (front) cutaway view of the abdominal organs of the digestive system. It shows the three main sections of the colon: the ascending colon, the transverse colon, and the descending colon. The ascending colon (on the right side of the body) plays a significant role in absorbing water and nutrients from food. The descending colon (on the left side of the body) stores and controls the evacuation of waste.

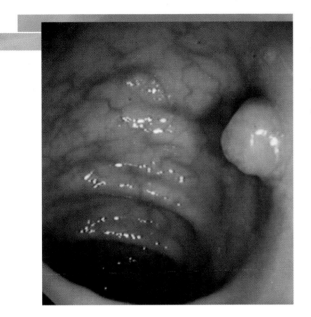

This medical image shows a non-cancerous polyp inside a patient's colon. Polyps often cause no symptoms. However, they can grow large enough to obstruct the flow of food through the intestine. When discovered, benign polyps are usually removed surgically to ensure that they don't become cancerous.

intestine, and stores the rest as waste. The waste eventually passes into the rectum and then out of the body through the anus.

Much of the knowledge of colon cancer has been learned by studying individuals afflicted with a condition known as familial adenomatous polyposis (FAP). It has long been known that colon cancer develops over a series of stages involving the growth of an adenomatous polyp, which is an excessive growth of the normal lining of the large intestine. These polyps are the premalignant lesions mentioned earlier. Over the course of eight to ten years, the polyp grows into a full-fledged cancerous tumor.

A normal human cell has forty-six chromosomes, threadlike structures found in the cell nucleus containing DNA and protein. It was discovered that patients suffering from FAP harbor a defect in a gene known as APC (or adenomatous polyposis coli). The APC gene, which is on chromosome 5, is supposed to govern the production of an enzyme that causes the degradation of a protein called beta-catenin. Beta-catenin,

FAMILIAL ADENOMATOUS POLYPOSIS (FAP)

Familial adenomatous polyposis (FAP) is a rare, inherited condition that primarily affects the large intestine. People with FAP develop hundreds of polyps called adenomas in their colons and rectums. Although FAP accounts for less than 1 percent of all colorectal cancer cases, it will almost certainly develop into colon cancer if it is not treated.

Children of individuals with FAP have a 50 percent risk of inheriting the mutated APC gene that leads to the disease. FAP usually does not skip generations, and it affects males and females of all races and ethnic groups. It is possible that a child may develop familial adenomatous polyposis even though neither parent has the condition. Mutations, or abnormalities, can occur within someone's APC gene when chromosome 5 is being transferred from parent to child. However, it is more likely that the mutation occurs after conception, during cell replication.

in turn, promotes the activation of an oncogene. So when the defective APC gene fails to effectively produce the enzyme necessary for breaking down beta-catenin, that excess beta-catenin activates the oncogene. Patients with FAP produce thousands of polyps, and have a 100 percent certainty of developing colon cancer unless some intervention is taken.

Other genetic anomalies associated with colon cancer have also been identified. Certain mutations on chromosome 18 lead to a loss of growth inhibitory factors. This makes the cell immune to stimuli designed to moderate its growth, which leads to uncontrolled cell division and the development of polyps. Also, an overproduction of the products of a gene known as Bcl2 leads to a loss of signals meant to prompt cell death.

WHO IS AT RISK?

Is it possible to predict who might have, or will develop, these genetic defects, and so be vulnerable to colon cancer? In a certain sense, it is. Age is a significant factor. The longer a person lives, the greater the chance he or she has of developing one of these mutations. The incidence of colon cancer rises after the age of forty. According to the National Cancer Institute, more than 90 percent of colon cancer diagnoses are in people over fifty years old. Colon cancer is extremely rare in children and young adults.

Diet is also a likely risk factor. A diet high in fat and alcohol, or low in folic acid, has been proven to raise the risk of colon cancer. It is believed that these diets promote the formation of molecules known as free radicals. Free radicals have a tendency to damage DNA, making the mutations that lead to cancer more likely. Other lifestyle indicators include smoking and physical inactivity.

A group of diseases known as inflammatory bowel disease (IBD) imparts a high risk of colon cancer. Inflammatory bowel disease has two variants: Crohn's disease and ulcerative colitis. In these conditions, persistent inflammation exists in the lining of the colon. As a result, the colon's tissues are constantly being damaged and repaired. As part of this process, the cells of the intestine are constantly dividing. Because of the sheer amount of DNA being manufactured, the likelihood of an error—a mutation—is very high. One of these mutations could turn the cell malignant, or cancerous.

Finally, the strongest predictor of colon cancer is having a family history of the disease, especially if the affected relative is a parent or sibling. This suggests that one of the mutations leading to colon cancer already exists in the family's genes, which are being passed from

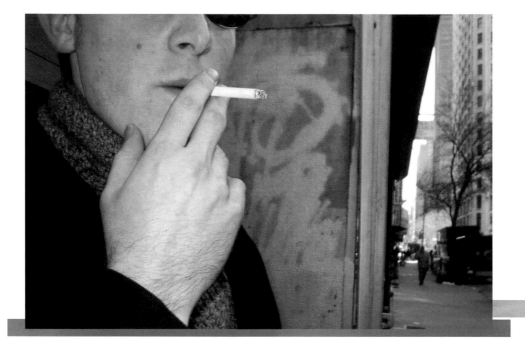

Cancer research shows that smokers and ex-smokers are more likely to die from colon cancer than people who have never smoked. Also, the more a person smokes the greater the risk he or she has of developing cancer. Smoking appears to cause colon cancer by limiting the cells' ability to repair damaged DNA.

generation to generation. Also, a person who has already had colon cancer may develop it a second time.

According to the American Gastroenterological Association, men and women of all racial groups are at an almost equal risk of developing colon cancer. However, the association observes that the survival rates appear to be lower for African Americans.

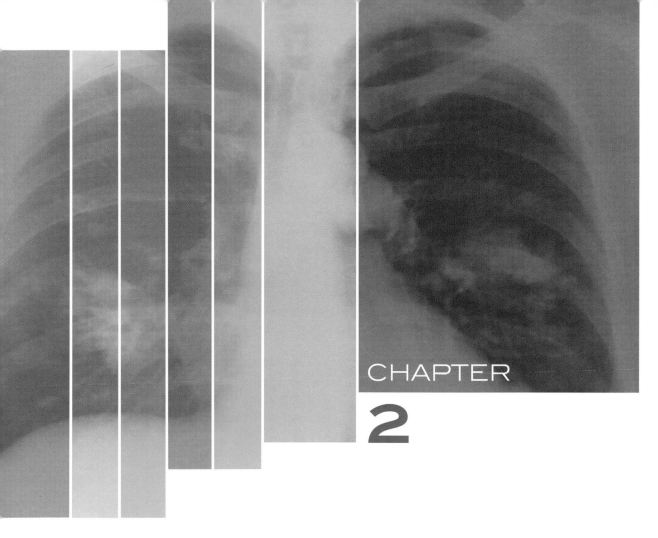

CHAPTER

2

COLON CANCER SCREENING AND STAGING

As we have discussed earlier, colon cancer evolves from a pre-malignant polyp, and it is possible to predict who is at risk for developing the disease. These two facts make it possible to prevent colon cancer by targeting screening measures to find premalignant polyps in at-risk people. This has been proven by a wealth of scientific information. Over the years, a number of screening tests to detect colon cancer have been developed. These include sigmoidoscopy, colonoscopy, virtual colonoscopy, and capsule endoscopy.

SIGMOIDOSCOPY AND COLONOSCOPY

A sigmoidoscopy is an internal examination of the lower colon. It is performed using a sigmoidoscope, which is a thin, lighted tube with a camera on one end. It is connected by fiber-optic wires to a TV monitor at the other end, allowing the physician to view the inside of the colon.

To have a sigmoidoscopy, the patient's lower colon must be empty. Therefore, the patient is given laxatives or enemas about two hours before the procedure to remove stool from the lower colon. After this preparation period, the sigmoidoscope is introduced through the rectum into the lower part of the large intestine. By so doing, the physician is able to view directly the lining of the last one-third of the colon, looking for polyps. The physician removes whatever polyps are found, thereby preventing them from becoming cancerous.

Several decades ago, this was quite adequate, as the vast majority of colon cancers and colon polyps developed in this one-third segment. In recent years, for reasons that are still being investigated, the occurrence of many polyps and cancers have migrated into the initial one-third of the colon, far out of reach of the sigmoidoscope. As a result, physicians now prefer to perform a colonoscopy, a procedure much like a sigmoidoscopy, but one that involves a longer instrument, allowing visualization of the entire length of the colon.

Both procedures are generally safe. The two major complications, major bleeding and perforation, or tearing, in the intestine, occur in fewer than one per 10,000 procedures. There may sometimes be reactions to the anesthetics used during the colonoscopy (sigmoidoscopies are done without anesthetics), but with the anesthetic agents available today, these reactions are rare. The largest concern about the procedure is a psychological one: people don't like the idea of inserting a large tube into their rectum. Quite possibly, this is the number one reason why these procedures are refused.

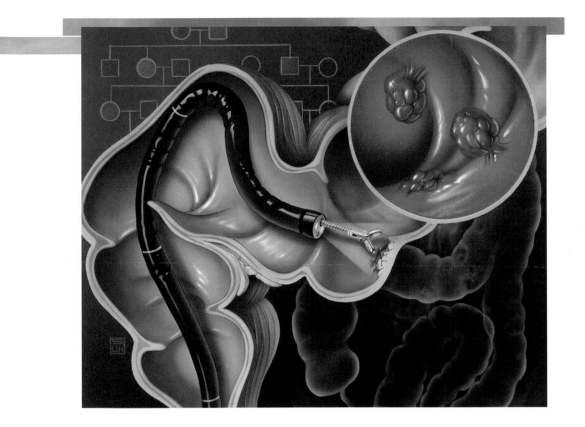

This illustration shows the removal of a polyp using a sigmoidoscope. In addition to detecting polyps, a sigmoidoscopy is used to find the cause of diarrhea, abdominal pain, and constipation. The procedure usually lasts between ten and twenty minutes. The scope is capable of blowing air into the colon, thereby inflating it and giving the physician a better view. The patient might feel pressure and a slight cramping in the lower abdomen. This will cease as soon as the air leaves the colon.

VIRTUAL COLONOSCOPY

Fortunately, within the past few years a new technique has been developed that more people find acceptable. This is called a virtual colonoscopy. In this procedure, a sophisticated computerized tomography (CT) machine uses X-rays and computer programs to create a

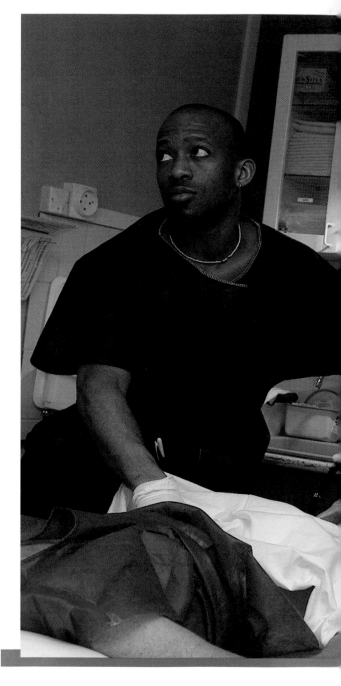

Two health care professionals look at the images on a monitor as they perform a colonoscopy. Colonoscopies allow the physician to look inside the entire large intestine for signs of cancer, as well as to diagnose the causes of unexplained changes in bowel habits. Typically, the procedure lasts between thirty and sixty minutes. The patient is usually given a sedative or pain medicine to keep him or her from feeling much discomfort during the exam.

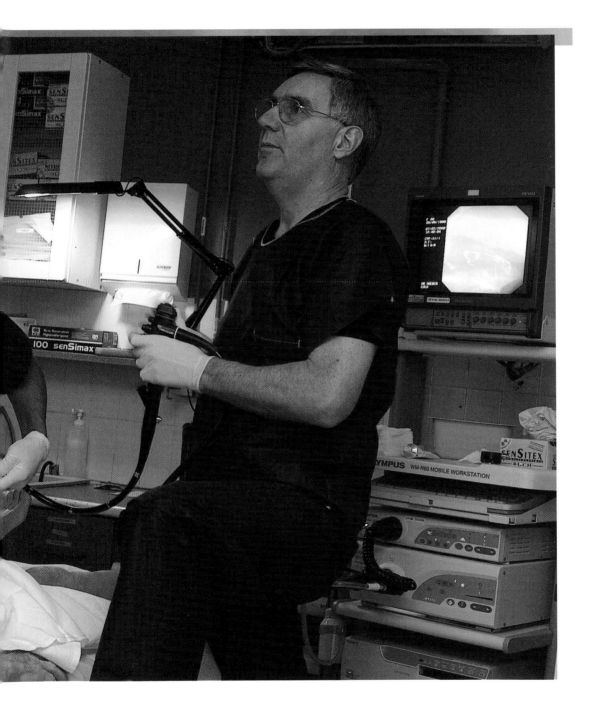

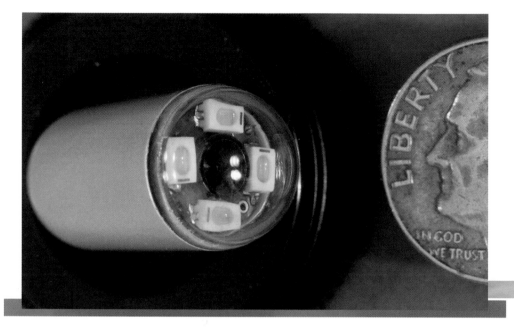

A miniature camera used in capsule endoscopy is placed alongside a dime in this photograph to highlight its tiny size. When swallowed, the pill-sized imaging device allows a patient to carry out normal activities during the examination, while images are sent to a receiver the patient wears.

detailed three-dimensional picture of the lining of the large intestine. The resolution of these pictures is quite good, and very small polyps and lesions can be seen. The main drawback is that if something suspicious is seen, the patient must undergo a real colonoscopy to have it removed, subjecting the patient to the risks and costs of two procedures instead of one. A virtual colonoscopy is not appropriate for individuals with a high likelihood of having polyps, as the chance that they would need to have a colonoscopy anyhow is almost certain. However, its use for screening for polyps in persons with average risk is acceptable, especially if such a patient would decline any other type of screening.

CAPSULE ENDOSCOPY

Another technology that is beginning to be used is capsule endoscopy. With capsule endoscopy, a patient swallows a capsule about the size of a multivitamin pill. The capsule contains a camera and a transmission device. As the capsule goes through the entire gastrointestinal system—from esophagus to rectum—the camera films the journey and transmits the images to a recording device the patient wears about his or her waist. At the end of the passage, the capsule is excreted with a bowel movement. The recording is then downloaded into a desktop computer for examination by a physician. Of course, much like the virtual colonoscopy, if something is seen that is suspicious, a real colonoscopy needs to be performed to examine and remove it. The process of removing and examining tissue from the body is known as a biopsy. The advantage of the capsule endoscopy is that areas of the gastrointestinal tract, previously nonvisible, can be evaluated.

STOOL SAMPLING

Physicians long have been able to test small samples of stool for microscopic amounts of blood. Most diseases of the intestinal tract at some point cause bleeding, most often in trace amounts, though sometimes more. Certain chemicals can be added to stool to detect the presence of hemoglobin, a major component of red blood cells. This technique is used to target patients requiring investigation with colonoscopy. More recently, tests have been developed to detect bits of abnormal DNA containing the mutations previously discussed. A positive test would alert the physician that a polyp or tumor was growing inside the patient's colon, and would prompt an urgent investigation.

A TRADITIONAL COLON CANCER SCREENING TEST RECEIVES A FAILING GRADE

One of the warning signs that a person may have colon cancer is hidden blood in the stool. Therefore, it seems to make sense for physicians to look for blood in the stool. For decades, doctors have been using the fecal occult blood test (FOBT) to screen average-risk individuals. However, a number of recent studies cast doubt on the effectiveness of this test in detecting colon cancer.

In one study, the researchers compared the results of a traditional fecal occult blood test using a single sample taken during a digital rectal exam (DRE)—where the doctor inserts a gloved finger into the patient's rectum—with the results of a test of six samples collected at home by the patient over the course of three days. Although the at-home FOBT was more effective than the single-sample test, both were found wanting. The study showed that the traditional FOBT failed to detect 95 percent of advanced-stage cancerous tumors. The at-home test missed the tumors 76 percent of the time.

A second study showed that approximately one-third of all physicians use the single-sample DRE blood test as their only method of screening for colon cancer. Considering the failure rate of that test, the implications are alarming. It suggests that many patients do not get the accurate results that they believe they are getting.

These findings will likely lead many cancer organizations and governmental health agencies to modify their recommendations regarding the fecal occult blood test. A colonoscopy remains the most highly regarded method for screening colon cancer.

SYMPTOMS OF COLON CANCER

While most often colon polyps and cancers are found as a result of a screening test, sometimes specific symptoms prompt an investigation. Irregular bowel habits are among the most common symptoms. As a polyp or tumor grows, it encroaches upon the lumen (hollow area) of the colon and impedes passage of stool. As such, constipation is a frequent symptom. A change in the normal appearance of stool is sometimes seen as well. As the stool is forced past an obstruction, it gets squeezed into a smaller diameter. As mentioned earlier, polyps and cancers typically bleed, and the sight of blood in a bowel movement is something that should prompt investigation. Sometimes the presence of symptoms will suggest the existence of metastatic disease, or cancer that has extended beyond the confines of the colon. Such symptoms include weight loss and ascites, which is the accumulation of fluid in the abdominal cavity.

STAGING COLON CANCER

Once colon cancer is diagnosed, it is important to determine if it has spread beyond the confines of the colon, as this will greatly influence therapy (treatment) and prognosis (chance of recovery). The process used to evaluate the extent to which cancer has spread to other parts of the body is known as staging. There are several staging systems. The most important is what is known as the Dukes stages. This staging system indicates how far from the inner surface of the colon the tumor has invaded.

The colon has several layers: the mucosa, the innermost layer, where polyps and cancers originate; the muscularis, which is the muscle layer that contracts to move contents onward; and the serosa, which is an outer covering. Surrounding the colon are groups of lymph nodes, collections of immune cells that filter the blood for invading organisms.

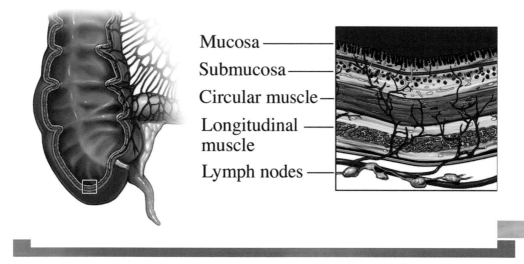

Mucosa
Submucosa
Circular muscle
Longitudinal muscle
Lymph nodes

This medical illustration shows the structure of the colon. The long hollow organ is lined on the inside with mucous membrane. There are two levels of mucous membrane: the mucosa and the submucosa. The muscle layers—circular and longitudinal—wrap around the entire length of the colon, helping food material move through to the rectum. The outer covering, the serosa, is surrounded by lymph nodes.

A colon cancer confined to the mucosa is termed a Dukes A stage; if it invades the muscularis but is still within the serosa, that is a Dukes B cancer. If tumor cells are found in nearby lymph nodes, that is a Dukes C, and if there is evidence of it being elsewhere, that is a Dukes D. It is important to determine the stage when considering treatment, for treatment directed locally will not be beneficial if the cancer has spread, as in the Dukes D stage, and therapy delivered to the entire body to treat a Dukes A lesion needlessly exposes the patient to the side effects of therapy. Moreover, the Dukes staging can give information important to survival. Ninety percent of patients diagnosed and treated for Dukes A

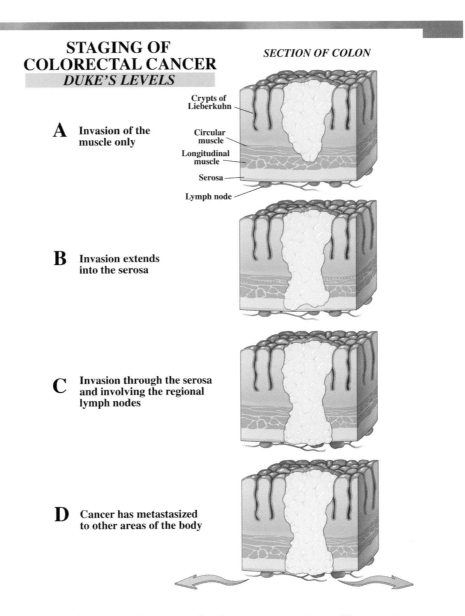

STAGING OF COLORECTAL CANCER
DUKE'S LEVELS

SECTION OF COLON

Crypts of Lieberkuhn

Circular muscle

Longitudinal muscle

Serosa

Lymph node

A Invasion of the muscle only

B Invasion extends into the serosa

C Invasion through the serosa and involving the regional lymph nodes

D Cancer has metastasized to other areas of the body

Staging is a crucial step in the care of colon cancer patients. The staging process helps physicians determine the best treatment options and also gives an indication of the patients' chances of survival. This illustration shows the extent of colon cancer for each level of the Dukes staging system.

CANCER STAGING SYSTEMS

The Dukes staging system is the classic staging system for colorectal cancer. It was developed by Sir C. E. Dukes, a British pathologist, in 1929. Although dated, the system is still widely used by physicians today. The original Dukes staging system had three stages: A, B, and C. It was modified in 1939 to include those tumors observed beyond the surgical margin.

The Dukes staging system is a site-specific system because it applies only to colorectal cancers. A more general cancer staging system for use in the United States was developed by the American Joint Committee on Cancer (AJCC) in the late 1950s. Called the AJCC/TNM system, it considers all aspects of cancer in terms of the size and invasiveness of the primary tumor (T), the presence or absence of tumors in regional lymph nodes (N), and the extent of the distant metastasis (M), or spread, of the tumor.

Between 1962 and 1974, the AJCC published a series of site-specific staging schemes. In 1998, it modified its staging system for colorectal cancer to correspond with the Dukes system. The AJCC/TNM staging system for colorectal cancer has five stages. Stage 0 indicates cancer that is limited to the innermost lining of the colon or rectum. Stages I through IV closely match Dukes stages A through D.

cancer are alive after five years. The five-year survival rate drops to 5 percent for Dukes D patients.

The spread of cancer from one part of the body to another is known as metastasis. Colon cancer cells generally spread, or metastasize, via the bloodstream. As such, typical sites of metastasis are the lungs and liver—two organs that in a sense act as filters, as the entirety of the blood volume passes through them. As part of the initial cancer evaluation, then, an X-ray of the chest and a CT scan of the liver are performed to examine those areas.

Another way that the spread of colon cancer is deduced is with a protein called the carcinoembryonic antigen (CEA). This protein is produced by some, though not all, colon cancers, and its level in the blood is somewhat correlated to the amount of cancer present in the body. It is useful to monitor CEA to document the response to therapy, as the level would be expected to diminish as the tumor is treated. It is also useful to monitor the patient for recurrence, as the level might rise if the tumor comes back after treatment.

In addition to doing chest X-rays, CT scans, and blood tests to check the CEA level, physicians may stage colorectal cancer by endoscopic ultrasound, a procedure in which an ultrasound probe is inserted into the rectum. This allows a physician to see into the layers of the intestine and so estimate the depth of tumor invasion. The ultrasound works similarly to the way radar does. Sounds are introduced into the tissue and recorded as they are bounced back, creating a picture similar to radar reports during a weather forecast.

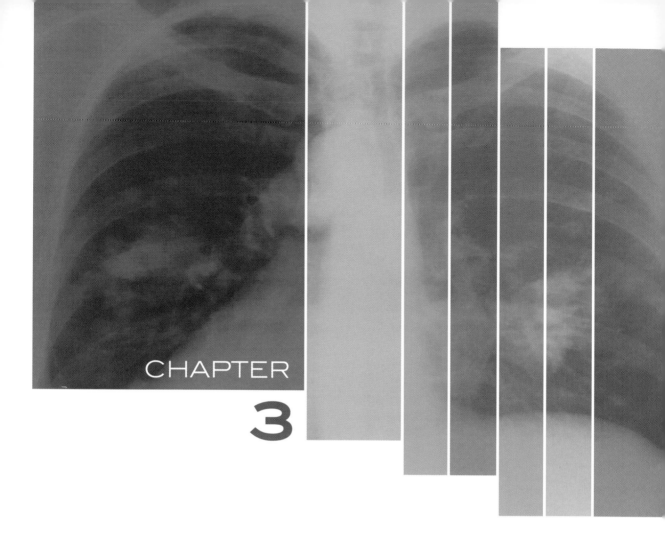

CHAPTER

3

TREATING COLON CANCER

The ultimate goal of any cancer therapy is to achieve a cure. Generally, cancer treatment depends on the size, location, and extent of the tumor, as well as the patient's general health. With colon cancer, this is best, and probably only, achieved with surgery. However, the treatment may also include chemotherapy, radiation therapy, or biological therapy. Sometimes, two or more forms of treatments are combined. As noted earlier, the selection of therapy is dictated by the extent of the tumor.

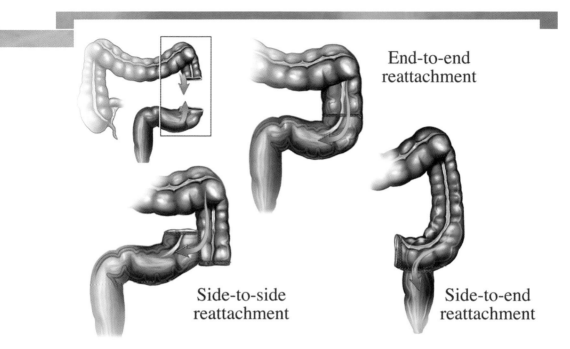

End-to-end
reattachment

Side-to-side
reattachment

Side-to-end
reattachment

This diagram illustrates the resection of a tumorous portion of a colon and three different techniques in reattaching the two ends of a resected colon. The reattachment can be done in a number of ways. A common method uses a stapling device that joins the two ends with stainless steel or titanium staples.

COLON CANCER SURGERY

If the cancer is confined to the colon wall, that is, if it is a Dukes A or Dukes B stage, it is possible that the tumor can be resected before it has spread, thereby achieving the cure. ("Resection" is the medical term for "removal by surgery.") During the resection, the surgeon will usually sample the surrounding tissues and lymph nodes as well. This allows a pathologist to look for evidence of microscopic spread beyond the colon, as this would greatly influence prognosis and further treatment. Typically, the segment of the colon that contains the tumor plus a few inches on either side is surgically removed. This procedure is called a hemicolectomy.

However, sometimes much more, perhaps even the entire colon, is removed. This would be the case if the patient had one of the familial polyposis syndromes discussed in chapter 1, where the risk of recurrence or a second tumor is so great that the resection is done in an attempt to prevent further cancers.

Depending on the site and size of the tumor, the surgeon may perform one of two procedures after resecting the tumor. The first is called an end-to-end anastomosis. This procedure involves reconnecting the healthy portions of the colon by sewing together the two loose ends of the intestine that resulted from the removal of the tumor.

Sometimes, however, the surgeon cannot reconnect the healthy portions of the colon. For example, the site of the tumor may be so low that its removal affects the rectal and anal muscles. When this occurs, the anal sphincter becomes damaged. The anal sphincter is a muscular valve over which one has conscious control to forestall a bowel movement until it is convenient. A damaged sphincter renders a patient incontinent. In other words, the patient can no longer control his or her bowel movements.

When the anal sphincter is damaged during a resection, the surgeon will create a colostomy, an opening into the colon from the outside of the body. This procedure entails sewing up the side of the colon below the tumor, in essence creating a "blind tube" (or nonfunctioning part of the colon) from the rectum upward. The other end, the one above the site of the tumor, is attached to a hole made through the skin of the abdominal wall. Stool is thus excreted through the opening—the colostomy—and is collected in a bag.

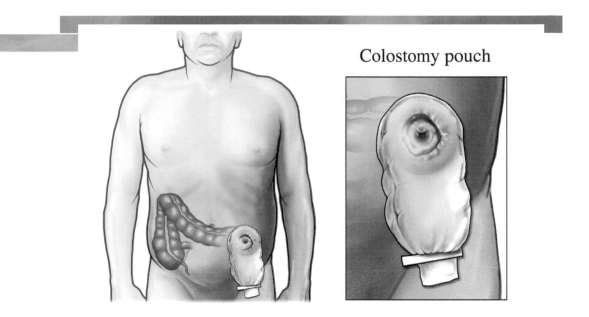

Colostomy pouch

A colostomy creates an opening to the exterior of the abdomen that operates as an artificial anus, through which the patient can pass waste material until the colon heals or other corrective surgery is performed. Patients who have had their rectums or anuses removed to treat cancer often require permanent colostomies.

Most colorectal cancer patients need only a temporary colostomy to allow the lower colon or rectum to heal. However, approximately 15 percent of them require a permanent colostomy.

Understandably, patients needing colon surgery are discouraged by the possibility of their needing a colostomy afterward. Fortunately, new technologies are being developed to prevent this need. One such development involves taking skeletal muscle—such as the type in our arms and legs under our conscious control—from one area and implanting it in the area of the anal sphincter. Controlled by electrodes embedded beneath the skin, this so-called neosphincter takes the place of the surgically damaged one. Researchers are currently exploring the

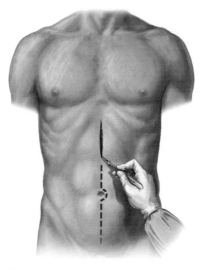

A. An incision is made in the abdomen.

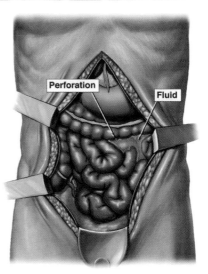

Perforation

Fluid

B. The abdominal cavity is exposed.

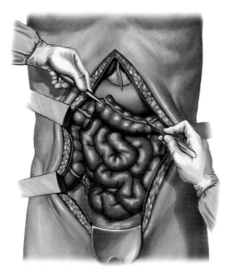

C. 12 to 15 centimeters of the transverse colon is removed.

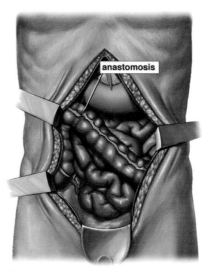

anastomosis

D. An anastomosis is performed with the remaining portion of the colon.

This medical illustration shows the extent of the incision, or cut, into the abdominal cavity during a laparotomy. A laparotomy is no longer the surgery of preference for treating colon cancer. However, sometimes a surgeon may perform the procedure to accurately diagnose a problem inside the abdomen. Colon cancer is one disease that may be discovered this way.

possibility of creating totally artificial sphincters, which can also be embedded.

LAPAROTOMY

The traditional approach to colon surgeries was via laparotomy. This entailed making a large incision from the breastbone downward, opening the entire abdominal cavity. The tumor was then found and resected. This surgery required a prolonged recovery period, was quite painful, and could result in various postoperative complications. Patients would often need to spend up to a week—sometimes even longer—in bed after the operation. This put the patient at risk of developing phlebitis, which is the inflammation of a vein, usually in the leg. Also, because of the large incision, infection and continued drainage from the wound were not uncommon. Moreover, prolonged inactivity put the patient at risk for pneumonia, bedsores, and muscle wasting.

If the tumor involved the rectum, additional surgery would be needed in the perineal area, that region in front of the anal opening. In addition to the complications described above, there is the added concern of rectal incontinence.

LAPAROSCOPIC COLECTOMIES

In recent years laparoscopic colectomies have revolutionized the surgical approach to treating colon cancer. The laparoscopic approach substantially reduced the postoperative problems—pain, lengthy recovery period, and risk of infection—associated with the laparatomic surgeries. In laparoscopic surgery, several small incisions, each less than an inch, are made in the abdominal wall, usually in the navel and to the sides. Next, carbon dioxide is pumped into the abdominal cavity, distending it (causing it to expand). Once this is done, an instrument with a camera on one end is introduced into the cavity through one of the small incisions. Video from inside the abdomen is projected

COLORECTAL CANCER SPECIALISTS

After diagnosing a patient with colon cancer, a primary care physician may refer him or her to a specialist. The medical professionals who are included in the staging and treatment of colorectal cancer include gastroenterologists, surgeons, medical oncologists, radiation oncologists, and pathologists.

A medical oncologist is a doctor who specializes in diagnosing and treating cancer using chemotherapy, hormonal therapy, and biological therapy. He or she often takes over the role of the main health care provider for cancer patients. As such, the medical oncologist often coordinates treatment provided by other specialists.

A gastroenterologist is a doctor who specializes in diseases of the digestive system. A radiation oncologist specializes in using radiation to treat cancer. A surgeon removes or repairs parts of the body by operating on a patient.

A patient who receives a colostomy during surgery is likely to see an enterostomal therapist, a health care professional who has been trained in the care of people with stomas. A stoma is a surgically created opening from an area inside the body to the outside, for example, a colostomy. The enterostomal therapist usually visits the patient before he or she undergoes surgery to explain what to expect. After surgery, this health care professional teaches the patient how to take care of the stoma.

Cancer patients typically don't have much contact with pathologists, who are doctors who identify diseases by studying cells and tissues under microscopes.

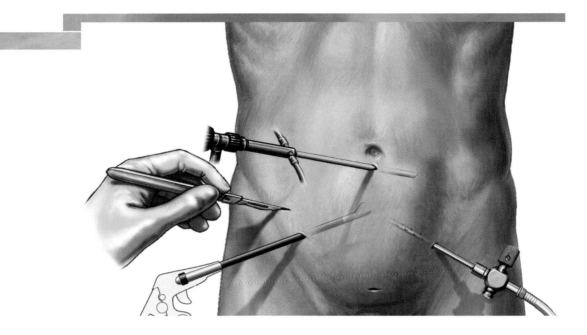

This illustration depicts the placement of three laparoscopic instruments into a patient's abdomen, as well as a surgeon's hand creating a fourth incision with a scalpel. In contrast to a laparotomy, laparoscopic surgery requires only small incisions to perform the operation. The development of laparoscopic surgery has made cancer treatment less painful and has reduced the period of recovery.

onto a TV screen. It is almost like seeing the inside of a basketball without cutting it open. Other surgical instruments, which are able to dissect, cut, and suture (sew), are put through the other incisions, and the surgeon operates them while watching where they are inside the abdomen via the video screen. In this way, the surgeon locates a cancerous tumor, cuts it out, and removes it through one of the incisions. It is much like playing a video game, and many of the same skills are required. In fact, during their training periods, surgeons practice on a simulator that resembles and operates like a video game. Once the surgery is complete, the instruments are removed, and the incisions are closed

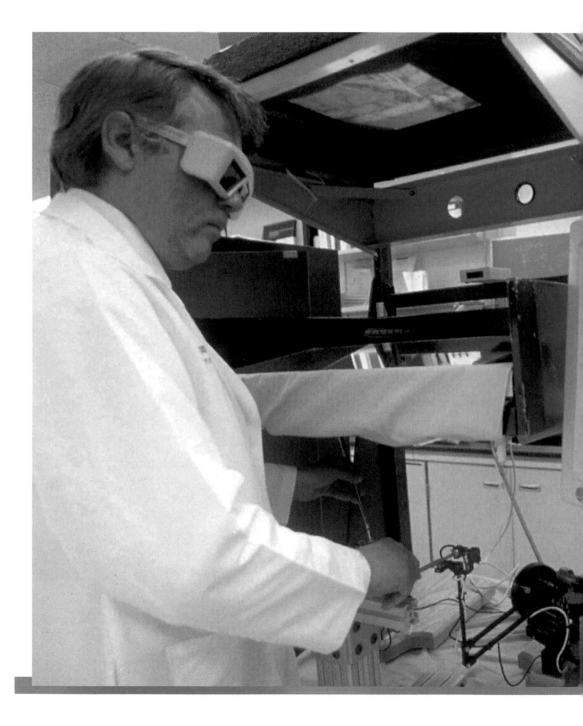

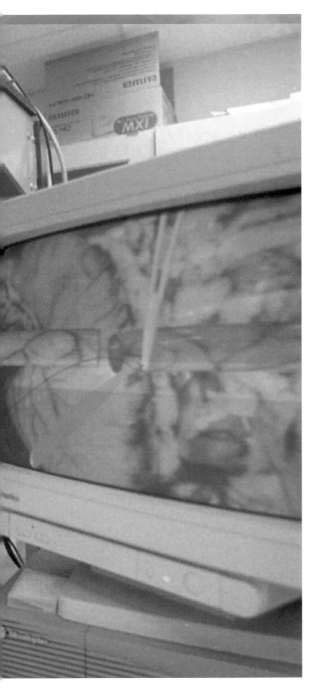

An engineer at the Milton S. Hershey Medical Center in Pennsylvania demonstrates the features of a Phantom machine, which is used to train medical students on various surgical procedures. The Phantom is not used in actual operations. However, the simulator combines computer graphics and virtual reality technology to give students a realistic experience in image-guided surgeries, such as the laparoscopic colectomy.

(sometimes with nothing more than a Band-Aid!). The bloodstream absorbs the carbon dioxide.

Because the amount of actual cutting in laparoscopic surgery is much less than during a laparotomy, the recovery period is considerably shorter. Patients are usually up and about within a day, and they go home a good deal earlier than with the other procedures. Moreover, because the surgical incisions are so tiny, the chances of infection are much lower.

SURGERY FOR RELIEF

Surgery also has a role for metastatic diseases—cancer beyond Dukes stages A and B—though not necessarily with the intention of curing them. Not infrequently, a tumor may be so large or positioned in such an awkward place that it causes obstruction of the intestine. This is very uncomfortable, with marked abdominal distension (swelling), and sometimes vomiting of stool. Should this occur, the physician may elect to perform surgery to try to relieve or bypass the obstruction somehow, simply to ease the discomfort. Sometimes, even with careful examination, a sole metastasis is found, perhaps in the liver or lung. In such an event, it is not unreasonable for the surgeon to attempt resection of this isolated lesion, in addition to the colon tumor, in an attempt to achieve a surgical cure.

CHEMOTHERAPY

For cancer that is only locally invasive, that is, limited to only the lymph nodes near the site of the original tumor, sometimes chemotherapy is given in what is termed an adjuvant therapy. With this strategy, chemotherapy is given before (in which case it is known as neoadjuvant) or after surgery, in hopes of improving the cure rate. By so doing, the chemotherapy is used in an attempt to destroy any remaining cells not removed by the operation. In addition, the neoadjuvant technique is

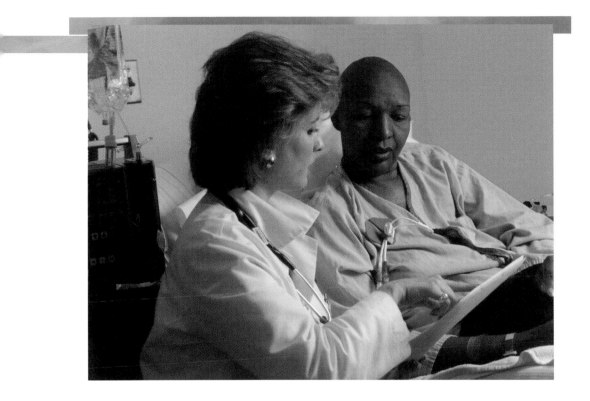

A health care professional consults with a female chemotherapy patient. Loss of hair is one of the most common, recognizable side effects of chemotherapy.

sometimes used to shrink the tumor mass, making the surgeon's job a bit easier.

DNA governs the growth of cells, and it is believed that mutations in the DNA structure might lead to change in a cell's function that in turn render it the ability to grow unchecked as a cancer. However, the integrity of the DNA in cancerous cells must be preserved to some degree. Otherwise, critical functions of the cell would cease and the cell would die. The ability to induce lethal mutations in DNA structure lies at the foundation of nonsurgical cancer treatment. By changing the structure of DNA, as with chemotherapy or radiation, physicians prevent the cell from reproducing properly, and the cell dies off. Chemotherapy, which is the practice of giving a patient chemicals in an attempt to treat a disease, is one way to accomplish this. Many types of tumors can be destroyed by using drugs that generally affect only cancer cells.

SIDE EFFECTS

Colon cancer treatment may lead to various side effects, of which patients are usually informed before the treatment begins. Side effects depend mainly on the type and extent of the treatment, and vary from patient to patient. In most instances, the side effects are temporary.

A patient who undergoes colon cancer surgery is likely to experience pain and discomfort in the area of operation during the first few days following the procedure. He or she may also feel tired or weak for a while, and may experience temporary constipation or diarrhea. The patient's health care team also monitors him or her for signs of bleeding or infection.

Patients who are given a colostomy during surgery may develop an irritation or infection around the opening. His or her doctor, nurse, or enterostomal therapist can teach the patient how to clean the area to reduce the risk of these side effects.

Chemotherapy affects normal cells as well as cancer cells. Reaction to chemotherapy depends on the specific drug or combination of drugs that is used and the dosage. Anticancer drugs generally affect those cells that divide rapidly, such as blood cells, cells in hair roots, and cells that line the digestive tract. Accordingly, the typical side effects of chemotherapy include infections, hair loss, loss of appetite, nausea, vomiting, diarrhea, and sores on the mouth and lips. Also, chemotherapy patients may bruise or bleed easily and feel weak and tired.

It is crucial for cancer patients to eat well during cancer treatment. Cancer patients need to get enough calories and proteins to maintain strength and a healthy weight. Eating well helps recovering cancer patients to have more energy and feel better. Understandably, many patients do not feel like eating when they are uncomfortable, tired, or experiencing side effects such as nausea, vomiting, diarrhea, or mouth sores. Fortunately, there are medicines to help relieve these side effects.

FOLLOW-UP CARE

After colon cancer surgery, the patient will be scheduled for regular follow-up visits with his or her gastroenterologist or oncologist. This follow-up care is very important, because it helps the doctor monitor the patient's recovery by checking to see if the cancer recurs, or comes back. Sometimes the disease returns because previously undetected cancer cells remained in the body after the malignant tumor was resected.

Doctors use a variety of tests to check for the recurrence or spread of cancer. Generally, these are the same set of tests used to diagnose cancer in the first place. They include colonoscopy; X-rays; CT scans; CEA test; and fecal occult blood tests.

It is widely recommended that a recovering colon cancer patient have a colonoscopy within three months after surgery, one year after surgery, and every three years after that. If the cancer does not recur within five years, it is considered to be cured.

THE FUTURE OF COLON CANCER TREATMENT

Chemotherapy is sometimes used in what is known as locoregional therapy, particularly for tumors that have spread to the liver or lung. It is possible, by using angiographic techniques—in which dye is injected into the bloodstream while X-rays are taken—to identify the one or two particular arteries responsible for delivering blood to the metastatic tumor. Once the artery is identified, a catheter (a tube) can be threaded into it, and a high concentration of the chemotherapy is delivered directly into the tumor. This technique has the advantage of using the chemicals to destroy the tumor while at the same time minimizing the exposure of normal tissues to the effects of the poisons.

EMBOLIZATION

Another interesting and new technique, also using the angiographic technique described above, is known as embolization. All tumor cells depend on a blood supply to continue to survive. Although "immortal," in a sense, they still require oxygen and other nutrients to grow. In fact, some types of cancers actually produce compounds that induce blood vessels to develop; in a sense, they produce their own supply line. After angiographically identifying the blood vessels responsible for keeping a tumor "alive," something, usually a metal coil, is placed in the blood vessel, causing it to close up with a large blood clot. Once this happens, the tumor is deprived of oxygen and other nutrients, and so dies. Another novel way of achieving this effect is with the use of antiangiogenesis factors. These are chemicals that induce the cancer cells *not* to make those compounds, impairing the cancer's ability to grow the blood vessels.

IMMUNOTHERAPY AND RADIOIMMUNOTHERAPY

The surface of every cell contains unique proteins that identify the cell to the body's immune system as being part of the body. This is how the immune system distinguishes normal cells from such invaders as bacteria and viruses. When cancer cells develop, these surface proteins sometimes become altered. These altered surface proteins can be isolated and purified, and produced in large quantities. They can then be injected into the body and act as a vaccine. The vaccine induces the immune system to recognize the colon cancer cells as foreign invaders, form antibodies against the cancer cells, and destroy them. This is known as immunotherapy.

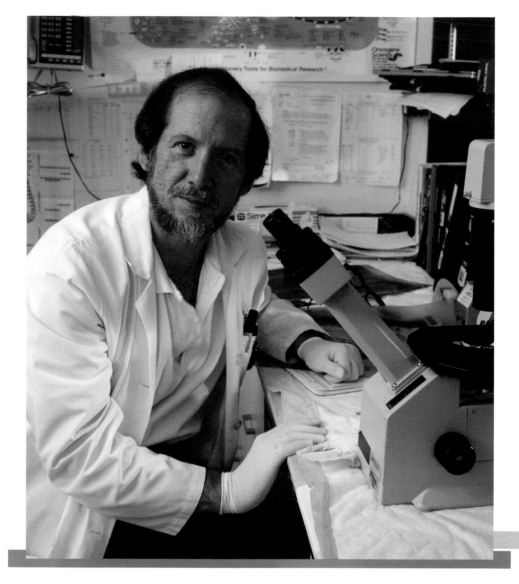

Dr. Bert Vogelstein of the Johns Hopkins University School of Medicine in Maryland is one of the world's leading colon cancer researchers. His research has led the world to understand that colon cancer is the result of a series of genetic mutations. He is currently working to improve a fecal DNA test to check for the mutation of colon cancer cells that may be passed in stool.

Furthermore, these antibodies can be isolated and used in a type of treatment known as radioimmunotherapy. In this process, the antibodies are attached to a radioactive compound and then reinjected into the patient. Because of the specificity of antibodies, they attach only to the cancer cells, delivering with them a lethal dose of radioactivity. This radioactivity damages the DNA of the cell, much the way chemotherapy would, as described earlier. Once the DNA is damaged, the cell cannot replicate properly. Because the antibodies attach only to the cancer cells, normal cells are left undamaged.

Some organs in the body are constantly regenerating themselves, replacing cells that die off with new cells. These are organs in a constant state of turnover. The skin, for example, is constantly flaking off in small bits, and new skin must develop. We bleed, and new blood cells must be formed. The colon, too, particularly the lining of the intestine, regenerates itself. For these regenerations to take place, there must exist a type of cell, a progenitor cell, which has the capacity to develop into whatever particular type of cell is needed. When the body needs a new gland cell, a progenitor cell evolves to fill that need. When more food-absorbing cells are needed, the progenitor cell has this potential, too. Because these progenitor cells have a near-limitless ability to turn themselves into something else, they can evolve into cancer. Indeed, it may be that cancer develops when one of these progenitor cells tries to evolve into a normal cell, but something happens along the way to alter its development and render it abnormal. A process known as differentiation therapy attempts to force the abnormal cell to continue its evolution to a normal cell, transforming it from a cancerous cell to a normal one.

BONE MARROW TRANSPLANTATION

Used for other cancers, particularly leukemia, bone marrow transplantation is finding a place in colon cancer treatment. First, a patient undergoes a matching process, in which another person with nearly

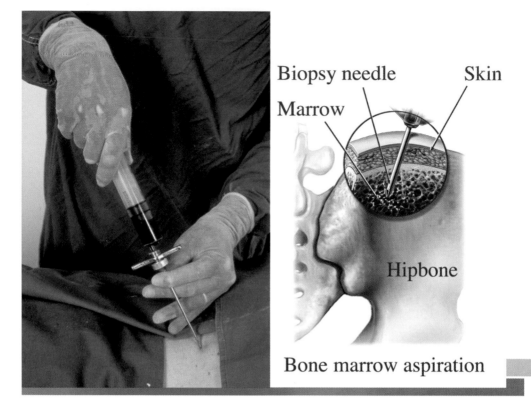

Biopsy needle   Skin

Marrow

Hipbone

Bone marrow aspiration

Bone marrow transplantation is used in colon cancer treatment to make it possible for patients to undergo high doses of chemotherapy and radiation therapy. This photograph and the accompanying illustration show the extraction of bone marrow from the hipbone of a donor.

identical genetic markers on cells of the immune system is found. This person, termed a bone marrow donor, allows some of his or her bone marrow to be harvested. The bone marrow, the hollow centers of some bones, is the place where the immune system cells are generated. In harvesting, some of this material is withdrawn using a large needle that punctures the bone. After this marrow is harvested from the donor, the cancer patient receives ultrahigh doses of chemotherapy. The doses are so high in fact, that the drugs kill not only the cancer cells, but cells everywhere in the body that are constantly regenerating, including those of the bone marrow. Left as such, the patient would surely die, as he or she has no capacity to rebuild his or her immune system, and would become susceptible to infection. However, the bone marrow, previously harvested from the donor, is infused into the cancer patient, hopefully restoring the immune system. The need to have identical genetic markers—as mentioned above—is important because otherwise, the "new" immune system would recognize the patient's body as foreign and go about destroying it.

CHAPTER
5

PREVENTION: THE BEST CURE

In recent years, the popular news media has given significant coverage to colon cancer in reporting on celebrities who have either been diagnosed with or have died of the disease. Many celebrities who are colon cancer patients, or have loved ones who are, have become engaged in public service campaigns aimed at encouraging people to get screened for the disease. Like the physicians and medical researchers who treat and study the disease, they emphasize a clear truth—colon cancer can be cured if detected early. More important, it can be prevented.

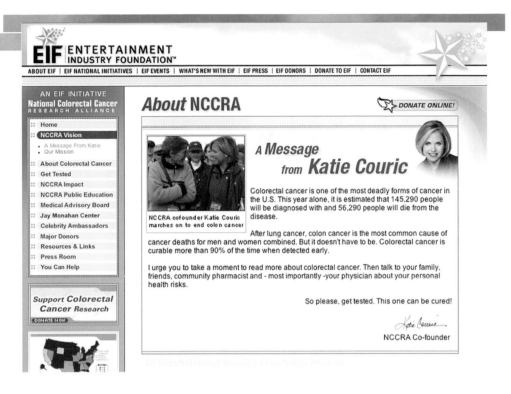

Television celebrity Katie Couric joined the fight against colon cancer after she lost her husband to the disease in 1997. She cofounded the National Colorectal Cancer Research Alliance (NCCRA) in March 2000 to help fund research in and increase public awareness of colon cancer. A screenshot of the foundation's Web site, featuring a message from the morning-show host, is pictured here.

As noted before, colon cancer is primarily an adult disease. The overwhelming majority (more than 90 percent) of colon cancer diagnoses are made in people over fifty years old. Accordingly, the National Cancer Institute recommends that everyone aged fifty or older be screened, and that those with a higher-than-average risk of colorectal cancer (for example, people with FAP) consult with their doctors about whether to undergo screening tests before the age of fifty.

MEAT AND COLORECTAL CANCER

In a study released by the American Cancer Society in January 2005, researchers show a strong link between a diet high in red and processed meats and the risk of developing colon cancer.

The researchers collected information on the meat consumption of nearly 150,000 people in 1982 and 1992, and tracked them to see which patients had developed colorectal cancer by 2001. They found that people who ate the most processed meat—which includes bacon, sausage, hot dogs, hams, and lunch meat—had twice the risk of developing colon cancer than those who ate the least. The study also showed that those who ate the most red meat—which includes burgers, meat loaf, beef, liver, and pork—had a 40 percent higher risk of developing rectal cancer. People who ate the highest quantity

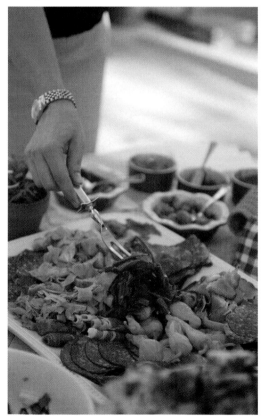

Red and processed meat remain mainstays in the American diet, despite warnings against eating too much of it. The average American eats about 65 pounds (30 kilograms) of beef each year.

of fish or poultry showed a 20 to 30 percent lower risk of developing the diseases.

It is still not clear which ingredient of meat triggers cancer, and further research needs to be conducted to confirm the American Cancer Society findings. Nevertheless, the evidence was strong enough for diet and cancer experts to recommend reducing the intake of red and processed meats and substituting them with poultry, fish, and beans.

COLON CANCER AND TEENS

It is true that the incidence of colon cancer is slight among children and young adults, but the lifestyle choices one makes during the teenage years can significantly influence one's chances of developing the disease in the future. For example, the evidence is quite clear that people who smoke are at a far greater risk of developing colon cancer than those who do not. Research also shows that teens who don't smoke are generally unlikely to become smokers in their adult years. Consequently, a teenager can reduce the likelihood of developing colon cancer (as well as other cancers, heart disease, and emphysema) later in life by resisting the peer pressure and temptation to smoke.

Of course, smoking is not the only risk factor for colon cancer. Other lifestyle choices such as diet and the level of one's physical activity can contribute to the development of colon cancer. Healthful eating habits that emphasize balanced meals and regular moderate or vigorous exercise decrease the likelihood of serious illnesses, including colon cancer. Specifically, it has been repeatedly demonstrated that obesity—often the result of poor eating habits and a sedentary lifestyle—poses a significant risk for developing colon cancer. Health

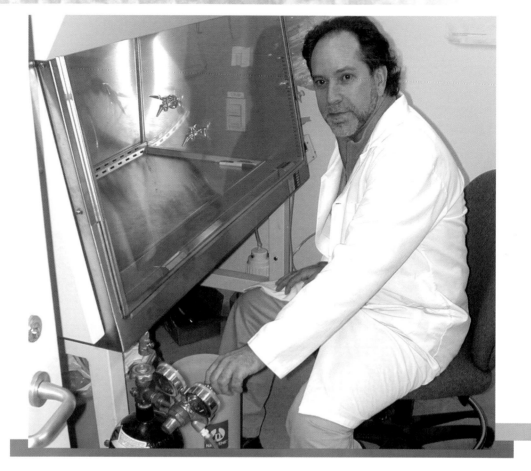

Dr. Daniel Rosenberg, pictured here in his lab at the University of Connecticut Health Center, is one of the leading colon cancer researchers in the United States. His current research involves trying to find a way to detect the earliest genetic signals that a person may develop colon cancer.

officials are concerned about the increasing incidence of obesity in the United States, especially among teens.

CONCLUSION

All across the world, medical researchers are studying new ways to prevent, detect, diagnose, and treat colon cancer. Also, many cancer patients are participating in clinical trials of various drugs and therapies. Some trials evaluate whether drugs used to treat other cancers could benefit colon cancer patients. Others study new drugs. One ongoing study being sponsored by the National Center for Complementary and Alternative Medicine (NCCAM) is investigating "the effect of acupuncture in reducing symptom distress in adults with advanced colon cancer."

As doctors work to discover new approaches to colon cancer, it is important to remember that colon cancer is preventable and, if detected early, curable. According to Dr. Randolph J. Hecht, associate clinical professor of medicine at University of California Los Angeles, School of Medicine, colorectal cancer "is essentially a cancer we can wipe out with education," as quoted in a January 22, 2001, *USA Today* article entitled "Dennis Franz Busts Colorectal Cancer." Dr. Hecht also said, "Every patient who gets colorectal cancer represents a lost opportunity." Dr. Hecht's message is clear: When it comes to colon cancer, prevention is the best cure.

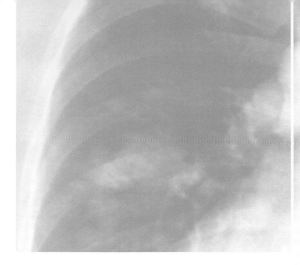

GLOSSARY

anesthetic Medication that reduces sensation, especially pain, and puts the patient in a sleeplike state.

anomaly A health condition not usually present in a healthy individual.

benign Not cancerous.

cancer Medical condition marked by an out-of-control growth and reproduction of abnormal cells.

capsule endoscopy An examination of the colon in which the patient swallows a capsule equipped with a camera and transmission device.

cell The smallest self-functioning unit in all living things.

chemotherapy Treatment with anticancer drugs.

colon The main part of the large intestine; part of the digestive system.

colon cancer Cancer that originates in the colon.

colonoscopy An examination of the colon with a flexible tube that has a light and a camera on one end.

colorectal cancer Cancer of the colon and rectum.

colostomy An opening into the colon from the outside of the body.

diagnosis Identification of a medical condition or disease through examination by a physician.

distend To expand.

DNA (deoxyribonucleic acid) The material within the nucleus of a cell that carries genetic information.

embolization The process by which an object is placed into a blood vessel, causing a blood clot to form.

enema A liquid placed inside the rectum to clear stool from the large intestine.

familial adenomatous polyposis A rare, inherited medical condition that causes hundreds of polyps to develop in the large intestine.

gene A unit of DNA that contains the information for a specific function; the functional unit of heredity.

immune cells Blood cells responsible for fighting bacteria, viruses, and other invaders of the body.

immunotherapy Type of therapy in which antibodies are used to destroy cancer cells.

laparoscopic colectomy Surgical procedure during which part of the large intestine is removed through a laparoscope.

laparotomy Surgical procedure during which a large incision is made in the abdominal wall, exposing the abdominal cavity.

lesion A tumor; mass of excess tissue that results from abnormal cell reproduction.

lymph Fluid that transports immune cells.

lymphatic system System of vessels carrying immune cells between lymph nodes.

lymph node Focal collection of immune cells.

malignant Cancerous.

metastasis The spread of cancer within the body.

mucosa The innermost layer of the colon.

muscularis The muscle layer of the colon.

oncogene A gene that makes a cell reproduce uncontrollably.

phlebitis Inflammation of a vein.

polyp A premalignant tumor of the intestines; a mass of excess tissue that results from abnormal cell reproduction.

prognosis The estimated outcome of a disease; the probability of the patient's recovery.

radioimmunotherapy A cancer treatment that combines radiation and immunotherapy.

rectum The last several inches of the large intestine that connects the colon and the anus.

resection The removal of part of an organ, such as cancerous tissue.

serosa The outer covering of the colon.

sigmoidoscopy An examination of the lower colon with a flexible lighted tube with a camera.

staging The process of determining the extent of a cancer.

suture A surgical sewing together.

therapy Treatment.

tumor A mass of excess tissue that results from abnormal cell reproduction.

virtual colonoscopy An examination of the colon by taking a series of X-rays called CT scans and using high-powered computer technology to view the X-ray images.

FOR MORE INFORMATION

American Cancer Society
(800) ACS-2345 (227-2345)
Web site: http://www.cancer.org

The American Gastroenterological Association
4930 Del Ray Avenue
Bethesda, MD 20814
(301) 654-2055
Web site: http://www.gastro.org/clinicalRes/brochures/fact-cc.html

American Institute for Cancer Research
1759 R Street NW
Washington, DC 20009
(800) 843-8114
Web site: http://www.aicr.org

Colorectal Cancer Network
P.O. Box 182
Kensington, MD 20895-0182
(301) 879-1500
Web site: http://www.colorectal-cancer.net

National Cancer Institute
(800) 4-CANCER (422-6237)
Web site: http://www.cancer.gov

WEB SITES

Due to the changing nature of Internet links, the Rosen Publishing Group, Inc., has developed an online list of Web sites related to the subject of this book. This site is updated regularly. Please use this link to access the list:

http://www.rosenlinks.com/cms/coca

FOR FURTHER READING

Clifford, Christine. *Our Family Has Cancer, Too!* Duluth, MN: Pfeifer-Hamilton Publishing, 1997.

Fromer, Margo Joan. *Surviving Childhood Cancer: A Guide for Families*. Oakland, CA: American Psychiatric Press, 1995.

Harpham, Wendy Schlessel. *Becky and the Worry Cup: A Children's Book About a Parent's Cancer*. New York, NY: HarperCollins, 1997.

Levin, B. *Colorectal Cancer: A Thorough and Compassionate Resource for Patients and Their Families*. New York, NY: American Cancer Society/Random House, 1999.

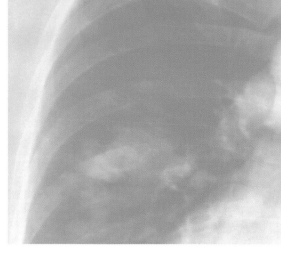

BIBLIOGRAPHY

Cirincione, Elizabeth. "Rectal Cancer." Emedicine.com. Retrieved November 2004 (http://www.emedicine.com/med/topic1994.htm).

El-Deiry, Wafik S. "Colon Cancer, Adenocarcinoma." Emedicine.com. Retrieved November 2004 (http://www.emedicine.com/med/topic413.htm).

El-Deiry, Wafik S. "Colon Polyps." Emedicine.com. Retrieved November 2004 (http://www.emedicine.com/med/topic414.htm).

Plickhardt, P. J. "Computed Tomographic Virtual Colonoscopy to Screen for Colorectal Neoplasia in Asymptomatic Adults." *New England Journal of Medicine*, December 4, 2003, Vol. 349, No. 23, pp. 2191–2200.

Podolsky, D. K. "Inflammatory Bowel Disease." *New England Journal of Medicine*, August 8, 2002, Vol. 347, No. 6, pp. 417–430.

Ransohoff, David F., and Robert S. Sandler. "Screening for Colorectal Cancer." *New England Journal of Medicine*, January 3, 2002, Vol. 346, No. 1, pp. 40–44.

Swaroop, Vege Santhi, and Mark V. Larson. "Colonoscopy as a
    Screening Test for Colorectal Cancer in Average-Risk Individuals."
    Mayo Clinic Proceedings, September 2002, Vol. 7, pp. 951–956.
The U.S. Preventive Services Task Force. "Screening for Colorectal
    Cancer: Recommendation and Rationale." *Annals of Internal
    Medicine*, July 16, 2002, Vol. 137, No. 2, pp. 129–131.

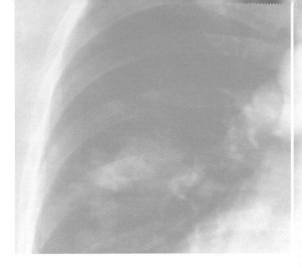

INDEX

ABOUT THE AUTHOR

Dr. Mark Stokes practices medicine in the North Shore Long Island Jewish Health System in New York, one of the nation's largest health systems. A graduate of SUNY-Stony Brook School of Medicine, he specializes in internal medicine. As a primary care doctor, he helps coordinate the diagnosis and care of cancer patients. He is also a lecturer and an associate program director for graduate medical education in the Department of Medicine at North Shore University Hospital.

PHOTO CREDITS

Designer: Evelyn Horovicz; Editor: Wayne Anderson